Disclaimer

Legal Notice:- The author of this book and the accompanying materials have used their best efforts in preparing the material. The author makes no representation or warranties with respect to the accuracy, applicability, fitness or completeness of the contents of this book. The information contained in this book is strictly for educational purposes. Therefore, if you wish to apply ideas contained in this book, you are taking full responsibility for your actions. The author disclaims any warranties (express or implied), merchantability, or fitness for any particular purpose. The author shall in no event be held liable to any party for any direct, indirect, punitive, special incidental or other consequential damages arising directly or indirectly from any use of this material, which is provided "as is", and without warranties.

Marijuana: 100 Benefits

By Richard Pabon

Table of Contents

Introduction:

This book was created to tell awareness on the real positive benefits of medical marijuana. I do not recommend the use of illegal marijuana.

Chapter 1: Marijuana

Marijuana (known as Cannabis, in the world of science) is a plant that many people use as a pleasurable drug and as a medicine. Its main compound, THC, is what causes the euphoric effect that many people experience when they use marijuana. Other than THC, there are 482 compounds in the plant, including cannabidiol, cannabinol, cannabigerol, and tetrahydrocannabivarin. These compounds are what give marijuana its unique properties.

Many people throughout history and today use marijuana to experience its euphoric effects. People who smoke or ingest it often report feeling happy, relaxed, and at peace. The most common side effects of marijuana use includes short-term memory loss, a decrease in motor skills, anxiety, red eyes, and dry mouth. Despite the legal controversies surrounding the drug, a 2004 study found that 4% of Americans admitted to using it.

Although marijuana has never killed anybody and it has many proven medical and environmental benefits, as you will soon read in this book, it is probably one of the most controversial topics in society today. It remains illegal in the majority of states and many people who could benefit from its medical properties are having a hard time getting to it in the first place.

From the 1950's onward, many have argued that marijuana was a "gateway" drug, meaning that it would encourage people who used it to try "harder" drugs. Although marijuana has a death rate of 0, it is still considered an illegal drug in the majority of the United States, despite its proven medical benefits. At the time of this writing, the only states who have approved marijuana for recreational use are Colorado and Washington State. 21 states have legalized medical marijuana and several states have decriminalized it (meaning that you cannot go to jail for possessing it), but there are still many states who carry harsh marijuana laws. For example, you can go to jail for 6 months and/or pay a $1,000 fine if you are caught with less than 50 grams in New Jersey.

Like any plant, there are several different varieties and strains of marijuana. The two most common strains of marijuana are cannabis Sativa and cannabis Indica. The different varieties of marijuana are created through cloning and seed breeding. Marijuana plants that grow in different regions are also considered as varieties. Marijuana plants are also grown for hemp, which is the fiber from the stem. Many people use hemp to manufacture every day products like paper, rope, and wood.

With over 5,000 different strains and the ability to be grown in almost any environment, marijuana has been around for centuries. The earliest signs of cannabis growth reach as far back as ancient China during 7,000 BC. Studies have shown that people in ancient China used marijuana for both medical and recreational purposes. Here is another fun yet intriguing fact: about six years ago, archeologists discovered *2 pounds* of cannabis plants in a 2,700-year old Shaman grave. Despite strict laws, modern civilizations followed in the footsteps of their ancestors. The Marijuana Tax Act of 1937 imposed a federal ban of recreational marijuana use.

In 1970, the federal government classified all forms of marijuana as a schedule I controlled substance, implying that it was just as dangerous as narcotics and served no use for medical purposes. However, that did not stop scientists from studying it and conducting experiments on it. Amazingly, extensive research over the years has proven that marijuana actually has many benefits to offer to peoples' health and the environment. Nearly 22,000 studies on marijuana have been published within the last couple of years. Scientists have concluded that it is not possible to overdose on it and it is non-toxic, making if the safest "drug" in the world, unlike its legal counterparts, tobacco and alcohol.

It was legal to grow hemp in the United States until 1937. George Washington and Thomas Jefferson even grew it and were in favor of it. During World War II, the United States government made the production of hemp legal so that it could be used to manufacture shoe materials, ropes, oils, and anything that was in short supply during that time period. Interestingly, it was not outlawed because it was considered dangerous—it was because it wood industry viewed it as a threat. To combat its growth, corporate companies claimed that it was a dangerous substance, that society had a marijuana

problem, and that hemp could cause people to become extremely violent. Today, it is only legal to grow hemp in Canada, Russia, China, India, and Europe.

Today, the debate over whether marijuana should be federally legalized is a hot one. In 2013, polls and surveys showed that the majority of Americans supported legalizing marijuana for the first time ever. At the time of this writing, President Barrack Obama is now looking into removing marijuana off the official list of dangerous drugs. It is currently considered a Schedule I drug. A Schedule I drug is a drug that has no accepted medical uses but a high abuse potential. Clearly, the placement of marijuana on Schedule I makes no sense, since there have been many medical breakthroughs. Though, as of now, marijuana stays classified with serious drugs such as LSD and Meth.

In this book, you will read about 100 benefits of marijuana to your health and to the environment, showing that marijuana has no place on Schedule I. You will also read about the different strains (Indica, Sativa, and hybrid) as well as learn the truth about the most common marijuana myths. Finally, you will see what some of the most famous people are saying about marijuana and you will learn about the death- rate of marijuana compared to tobacco, alcohol, and pharmaceutical drugs.

Chapter 2: Marijuana Strains (Indica, Sativa, Hybrid)

As you know, there are two main categories of marijuana plants: cannabis Indica and cannabis Sativa. Since people all over the world grow marijuana, through cloning, seed breeding, and region-breeding, many different strains have been created. Those strains are known as Hybrid strains. There are over 5,000 different varieties of marijuana in the world today. Although this book cannot touch upon each one, this chapter will introduce you to some of the most popular strains under each main category.

Cannabis Indica Strains

OG Kush: OG Kush stands for "Original Gangster" Kush and originates from the San Fernando Valley in LA. Best harvested in mid-September, many people consider OG Kush to be one of the strongest strains of Indica because of its high THC count. This type of marijuana is best grown indoors, under hydroponic conditions. The side effects of this strain include an increased heart rate and physical stimulation.

Blueberry: Blueberry is a combination of strains from Indica and Sativa, but since it its 80% Indica, it is considered an Indica strain. Best harvested in mid-October, Blueberry gets its name from its flavor and the blue color that each plant possesses. When grown outdoors, Blueberry keeps most of its flavor, a very fruity, blueberry-like taste. Blueberry is also best known for its long lasting euphoric effect. Blueberry is such an excellent strain of marijuana that it has won multiple prizes and nominations.

LA Confidential: LA Confidential is similar to OG Kush in origins and structure. Most popular in the 90s, its name was coined by several famous rappers through their songs. LA Confidential is said to put smokers in a hazy, trip-like state. This strain can be grown both indoors and outdoors. When this strain is close to harvest, the leaves often turn a dark, black color.

Bubba Kush: Bubba Kush is an Indica plant that was created when seeds from North Carolina were mixed with a pure Kush plant. This strain has made its way from the west coast to the east coast and is considered a classic. It is not as pure as OG Kush, Bubba Kush has a sweet taste and odor. It takes about 7 to 9 weeks to grow this strain. The effects of Bubba Kush include "the munchies" and laziness.

Northern Lights: Northern Lights is a strain that is one of the most famous types of cannabis Indica. Indoors, it can be grown in just six weeks. Each Northern Lights plants grows to about four or five feet and possesses a sweet/spicy taste. The effects of Northern Lights are relaxing and comfortable. In 1990, Northern Lights won the High Times Cannabis Cup.

Purple Kush: Purple Kush is a medical strain of marijuana that originated in California. Since it is a cloned strain, you can find it in states other than California. Many patients who receive this strain for medical purposes use it to treat depression, inflammation, and pain. Mostly grown indoors, this strain can grow to about two or three feet tall. Once its buds are ripe, the leaves turn from green to purple.

Cannabis Sativa Strains

Sour Diesel: Sour Diesel is a strain of marijuana that has a strong growing odor and a sour, lemon-like taste. With origins in Mexico, sour diesel is a tall, green plant that can reach up to six feet. The leaves of sour diesel can be pink and purple. The side effects of sour diesel include taking the user into a spiritual-like state, with euphoric, perspective-changing vibes. Sour diesel is a good strain for relieving chronic depression.

Trainwreck: Trainwreck is a pure Sativa strain that is commonly used for both medical and recreational purposes. Trainwreck is known for its most unique smell and taste. With possible origins in North Carolina, Trainwreck gives its users a clear-headed effect. Many patients use it to relieve muscle tension. Many people like to smoke it after playing extreme sports that put strain on the muscles. Grown indoors, it takes about eight weeks to produce Trainwreck. It can also be grown outdoors in early October.

Blue Dream: Blue Dream is a strain of marijuana from Northern California where the strains Blueberry and Haze were mixed together. Blue Dream has dense, puffy buds that have orange hairs and blue/purple hues. Some describe its taste as tropical or sweet and spicy. The effects of Blue

Dream include a sense of focus, calmness, and relaxation. Many people chose to use Blue Dream for marijuana food products. Its THC potency is 17%.

Purple Haze: Purple Haze became a common name to both smokers and non-smokers alike during the 60's and 70's hippie phase. Full of flavor, Purple Haze is a classic strain of marijuana. Purple Haze grows tall and possesses purple buds. This strain can be grown both indoors and outdoors. Its taste is smooth and its high is uplifting and euphoric. Many smokers use this strain to smoke socially and medical marijuana patients prefer it for relieving anxiety and muscle tension.

Strawberry Cough: Strawberry Cough is an indoor grown marijuana strain that has a sweet and creamy berry taste. Growing up to three feet tall, Strawberry Cough takes about two months to grow. It grows exceptionally well in greenhouses. Many people like to smoke Strawberry Cough to fight depression, as it gives its user an uplifting, energetic high.

Casey Jones: Casey Jones is a strain of marijuana that comes with a heavy high and a flavor of sweetness. Named after an engineer of one of the most famous train wrecks, this strain takes about eight weeks to grow. It has a citric/sweet/sour taste and a long-lasting high. Its effects can include feeling strongly connected to others and invoking a sense of creativity.

Hybrid Strains

Hybrid strains are strains that contain a little bit of both cannabis Indica and cannabis Sativa. Cannabis breeders like to breed the best strains to get the best hybrid results. Here are some of the most popular hybrid strains of marijuana:

White Widow: White Widow is a hybrid strain that contains 60% Sativa and 40% Indica. Since its first appearance in 1995, this strain has become a classic and a favorite among those who use marijuana. It was originally created by the Greenhouse Seed Company. When smoked, White Widow has a fruity, flowery taste and gives users a warm, trippy feeling. Best grown indoors, White Widow took the High Times Cannabis Cup in 1995.

AK-47: AK-47 is a hybrid strain that contains 65% Sativa and 35% Indica. Originally created in 1992 by Serious Seeds, AK-47 has a skunk-like scent and a sweet, floral taste. Best grown indoors, AK-47 grows tall and has a quick flowering time. The effects of AK-47 include an immediate, long-lasting buzz that is perfect for social smoking. The THC content of AK-47 is 20%.

Jack Herer: Jack Herer is a hybrid strain grown by Sensi Seeds. It possess a skunk-like scent and is best grown in dry climates, like California or Spain. In any other place in the world, Jack Herer must be grown inside. The effects of Jack Herer include an uplifting, visually enhanced high.

Lemon Skunk: Lemon Skunk is a hybrid strain that is 60% Sativa and 40% Indica. Taking eight to nine weeks to grow, Lemon Skunk possesses a fruity, citrus taste. When smoked, Lemon Skunk is known to heighten the senses, invoke mental reflection, and heightened perception. It can also induce an appetite. Lemon Skunk has won various awards between 2007 and 2009.

Master Kush: Master Kush is a hybrid strain created by Nirvana Seeds. Originally named High-Rise, Master Kush possesses no smell while growing and is almost tasteless when smoked. It is more like a smooth smoke that is easy on the lungs. It gives off a relaxing, happy buzz. This strain won the High Times Cannabis Cup two years in a row (1992 and 1993).

NYC Diesel: NYC Diesel is a 60% Sativa 40% Indica hybrid strain created by Soma Seeds. It can be grown indoors or in tropical climates and each plant can produce 100 grams. Reaching as high as 12 feet tall, NYC Diesel is good for invoking creativity during the day. It won three cannabis cups so far.

Chapter 3: 100 Benefits of Marijuana on Yourself and Your Environment

Now that you have learned a little about marijuana, its history, and the different types of strains and their effects, you will now learn about the various benefits that this plant has on health, the environment, and the economy. With over 100 benefits, it seems that marijuana can help almost anybody with something.

Most Useful Plant. Out of all the plants able to be grown in the world, the cannabis plant creates more food, fiber, and medicine than any other. It can be grown in almost any environment, making it a renewable resource. It has no negative impacts on the environment or on a person's health.

Over 5,000 Varieties. Although Chapter 2 touched on some of the most popular strains, there are over 5,000 varieties of marijuana worldwide. Each strain has its strengths and weaknesses and induce different effects on different people. Some strains are good for beating depression and other strains are good for calming violence. Every strain is great for helping with something, whether the environment, the economy, or your health.

Mood enhancer. Marijuana is a proven mood enhancer. While Indica strains are best for getting you into a relaxed, ready for bed mood, Sativa strains are best for acquiring a burst of energy. Many people report that engaging in sexual relations while high feel more connected to each other. Different strains induce different moods.

Source of Amino and Fatty Acids. Cannabis and hemp seeds contain important amino and fatty acids that people use in their diets every day. What makes marijuana unique is that it is the only plant that can produce digestible forms of these nutrients.

Nutritional Oil. Hemp seeds can be processed into nutritional oil that contains almost the exact amount of nutrients that the human body requires. Hemp seed oil contains a 3:1 ratio of omega-6 and omega-3 acids, which is enough to balance your body.

Paper Products. Hemp can be used to produce recyclable paper products such as stationary, computer paper, journals, cardboard, and even tampons. When hemp is used to make paper, rather than trees, there is no need to cut down more trees.

General Pain Relief. Marijuana is a popular remedy for general pain relief. Some studies have found that smoking marijuana for pain relief is just as effective as using a mild narcotic such as codeine. Researchers found that those who smoked a strong form of marijuana were able to tolerate pain for at least 12 seconds longer than those who took a placebo pill-form drug.

Increase Appetite. Some strains of marijuana are known to induce one's appetite after smoking. This side effect is commonly known as "the munchies." In medical purposes, marijuana can be used in a healthy way to induce the appetite in those who suffer from illnesses that may suffer from loss of appetite.

Prevents Nausea and Vomiting. Studies have shown that marijuana can be effective against the nausea and vomiting that can follow chemotherapy, certain surgeries, treatments for AIDS, and more. By suppressing this side effect it would also prevent against unhealthy weight loss.

Helps Treat Glaucoma. Marijuana has been shown to help slow or prevent glaucoma, a disease that can eventually lead to blindness. A handful of studies has shown that marijuana can take pressure off the eyes, which can help offset glaucoma.

Protects Against Cancer. Current research suggests that marijuana may be good for treating certain types of cancer, including breast cancer, brain cancer, prostate cancer, and lung cancer. Cancer patients report it being most helpful for treating chemotherapy side effects. Researchers around the world are currently studying marijuana's effect on cancer for further development.

Relieves Tourette's Syndrome Side Effects. Clinical studies have shown that marijuana can be effective against the side effects from Tourette's Syndrome. Researchers found that THC can help decrease the number of tics one has and it can also decrease one's obsessive compulsive behavior.

Helps Decrease Seizures. There have been several studies on animals and one experimental study on humans on the topic of marijuana and seizures. In the one human study, the results showed that patients who were exposed to THC showed a decline in the activities of seizures. Many people who live in countries in which marijuana is legal also report decreases in seizures after smoking marijuana.

Blocks Migraine Pain. The chemicals in marijuana and the chemicals in your brain can act together to block your brain's pain receptors, thus preventing the pain that is associated with migraines. It makes a good alternative to migraine medications that bring on negative side effects.

Relieves Multiple Sclerosis Symptoms. When taken in spray or pill form, marijuana has been found effective in relieving the symptoms of Multiple Sclerosis patients. Studies suggest that the cannabinoids in each plant, rather than the THC content, is what helps relieve the symptoms.

ADD/ADHD Treatment. Though the research is low right now, many doctors are in favor of using marijuana to treat ADD/ADHD instead of the traditional stimulant drugs, since marijuana is not addictive and is therefore much safer, especially for children. The study that found the strongest evidence that marijuana can treat these disorders found that marijuana can help stimulate certain counteractive chemicals in the brain.

Can Relieve Crohn's Disease. A few recent, small studies have shown that marijuana can help reduce the side effects of Crohn's Disease, also know as Inflammatory Bowel Disease. One of the studies found the marijuana caused the disease to go into remission. While researchers were unable to pinpoint the specific reasons as to how marijuana was able to combat Crohn's, they were able to confirm that the chemicals were able to relieve inflammation and nausea.

Slows Development of Alzheimer's Disease.
According to a professor of neurology at Ohio State
University, small doses of marijuana can help slow
the development of Alzheimer's Disease. This is
because marijuana acts as a anti-inflammatory
medicine and THC can directly affect the cycle of
Alzheimer's.

Can Relieve PMS. Marijuana can be used as an
alternative to painkillers to treat the symptoms that
many women experience during PMS, including
cramps, anxiety, and headaches. It is also a good
alternative to anti-depressants because anti-
depressants can take several days to kick in, while
marijuana can treat the symptoms immediately.

Does Not Take a Toll on Lung Health. Recent
studies have shown that long-term marijuana
smoking does not have any negative impacts on
your lung health as smoking does. Researchers
discovered this by asking participants to do a lung
test in which they measure how much air each
person can push out after taking a deep breath.
Interestingly, researchers found that those who
smoke marijuana can deliver more air than a person
who smokes tobacco.

Can Lessen Pain From Muscle Spasms. Research
has shown that marijuana can help relieve the pain
from muscle spasms, especially when an extract
spray is used. A majority of people who suffer
from muscle spasms have actually said that
marijuana has lessened the pain and has kept them
alive.

More Tax Revenue Potential. Legal marijuana has been bringing Washington State additional tax revenue through its sales. Experts estimate that it could bring the state as much of $500 billion. These tax dollars could go toward public health, healthcare costs, and health insurance costs.

Can Help Increase State Budget Savings. Legal marijuana can help states save additional money after accounting for tax revenue and less enforcement costs. The additional state income can help local governments give their residents a better quality of life.

Can Help Save On Enforcement Costs. Studies show that if marijuana was legalized federally, it would save the government about $13.7 billion dollars on enforcing the laws against it. Since one cannot overdose on marijuana, this would allow police forces to focus on enforcing laws against drugs that can hurt people.

Can Prevent Deforestation. Hemp can be used to create paper. One acre of hemp can produce quadruple the amount of paper than an acre of trees. This would save on the environment, as newspapers, writing paper, cardboard, and even tampons can be made from it.

Can Create Less Pollution. When hemp is used to make paper, it doesn't require as much pollutants or toxic chemicals, which can take a great weight off of the environment. Currently, many industrial manufacturers are polluting the air with the various chemicals and pollutants that come off as a byproduct of their products.

Serves As Replacement For Cotton. Hemp can be used as an alternative to cotton. Since cotton only grows under warm climate conditions, it takes a lot of water to harvest it. Hemp does not take up as much water and it can be grown anywhere.

Eliminates Pesticides. Hemp does not attract pests or insects, so it reduces the need to spray pesticides on the environment. Farmers often spray their crops and farmlands with chemical pesticides that are harmful both to the environment and your health.

Serves as a Wood Substitute. Hemp can also serve as a wood substitute. It is stronger than wood made from trees and again, does not require the destruction off too many trees. Using a hemp wood substitute can also save on the construction costs.

Is a Renewable Resource. Many products made from hemp are biodegradable, non-toxic, and renewable, leaving a positive, lasting impact on the environment. Resources that are nonrenewable often take up space in landfills and leave a toxic aftermath on the land and soil.

Hepatitis C Treatment. Researchers believe that marijuana can ease the side effects from Hepatitis C treatments and can help those who suffer from it overcome the disease. Some researchers also believe that marijuana can act as an antiviral medicine.

Reduces Suicide Rates. Marijuana is believed to reduce general suicide rates by 5% and by 10% among young men. Researchers came to this conclusion by analyzing the suicide rates in states where medical marijuana was legal and states where it was illegal. They believe that marijuana can help people cope with stress and other negative life events.

Relieves Arthritis. Marijuana is great for relieving arthritis because it serve as an anti-inflammatory medicine and it can relieve pain in the joints at the same time. A 2005 study showed that THC was able to help people with arthritis sleep better, lessen pain, and reduce progression of arthritis.

Boosts Metabolism. Some studies have revealed that smoking marijuana can help boost your metabolism. Although marijuana is known to increase one's appetite, it also increases ones heart rate, which can help burn more calories.

Relieves Lupus Symptoms. Similar to arthritis, marijuana is also known to help treat Lupus, another autoimmune disease. Many people who suffer from Lupus have reported that they prefer using marijuana to treat their symptoms and relieve pain over prescription drugs due to the negative side effects that follow many of them.

Inspires Creativity. Many famous people, such as Louie Armstrong, Jack Nicholson, and even Shakespeare have attributed their creativity to marijuana. Scientific evidence has recently shown that marijuana does, indeed, stimulate creativity in the brain. It also helps more blood go to the right side of the brain, which is responsible for creative thoughts.

Soothes Parkinson's Disease. Studies have found that marijuana has helped those who suffer from

Parkinson's Disease ease their tremors and sleep better. These studies were conducted in Israel, where it is commonplace to give marijuana to help those who suffer from Parkinson's.

Helps Veterans Cope with PTSD. It has been found that marijuana can help veterans, or anybody who suffers from Post-Traumatic Stress Disorder, learn how to forget the stimuli and/or noises that trigger their bad memories. For the best results, a low to medium dose of marijuana should be smoked to help invoke forgetting the bad memories.

Aids in Stroke Recovery. Brain damage, which usually occurs after a stroke, may be avoided with marijuana. New studies have found that certain chemicals in the plant can help reduce the size of the part of the brain that was hit hardest by the stroke. The cannabinoids found in marijuana can also help improve the function of the brain once the stroke has already occurred.

Helps Prevent Brain Trauma. Amidst all of the studies that have suggested that marijuana can actually cause brain damage, new leads believe that it can actually help prevent future brain trauma. This is because when low doses of THC impact the brain, it actually prepares the brain to guard itself against really bad damage. It is similar to getting a shot to let your body build up resistance to a certain disease.

Could Prevent HIV From Spreading. Researchers believe that the THC in marijuana can help block the disease HIV from spreading into the brain. It can also cause a slow in the duplication of infected cells. Though THC cannot cure HIV, it can stop people from suffering from memory loss and the ability to speak.

Helps Lower Insulin Levels. Since a couple of population studies showed that those who smoked marijuana smaller rates of diabetes and obesity, studies looked at what kind of effect marijuana has on blood sugar levels. Although studies are still being conducted to find the exact relationship between marijuana and low blood sugar levels, researchers believe that that cannabinoids in the plant cause the brain to release chemicals that help the body regulate blood sugar.

Stimulates Spirituality. Marijuana is known to help people focus and think in a way in which their conscious is altered. It can open one's mind up to learn new aspects of personal growth, peace, and love. It also helps people feel connected to each other so that they can create new things together.

Requires Less Pesticides and Energy. To grow marijuana, it does not require as much energy and pesticides that it takes to grow other plants. This is good for the environment because it doesn't expose the land to harmful chemicals and it saves on energy that can be used elsewhere.

Saves on Soil. Hemp does not put a lot of strain on the soil it grows in and does not need as much fertilizer as other plants do. Using less fertilizer means that there will not be as much water pollution due to water runoff.

Source of Renewable Energy. Hemp produces enough biomass to create a clean-burning alcohol fuel or coal that does not contain sulfur. Experts believe that hemp could account for 100% of energy in the United States if it was grown more.

Keeps Kids Away From Harmful Substances. According to the national institute of drug abuse, more and more teenagers are picking to use marijuana over alcohol and tobacco, which can lower their chances of developing lung cancer or liver disease. Marijuana is also safer them prescription drugs and painkillers, most of which are addicting and responsible for many overdoses.

Can Fight Anorexia. Strains of marijuana that induce "the munchies", otherwise known as an appetite, can help people who are underweight. The mother of one ten-year old boy with aggression and eating problems due to autism experimented by giving him marijuana brownies. She discovered that the brownies made him calmer and he began to eat different foods.

Could Reduce Traffic Accidents. Although there is no concrete explanation to this theory, one recent study has found that there are less traffic accidents in states that have legalized marijuana verses states that have not. Some people speculate that it's because people who are high drive safer because they have to concentrate on the road but there are no definite facts yet.

Has No Death Rate. Compared to alcohol, tobacco, pharmaceuticals, and other illegal drugs, marijuana continues to have a death rate of zero. Additionally, studies have shown that marijuana smokers are likely to live just as long as non-marijuana smokers.

Shrinks Tumors. In the year 2000, researchers discovered that they were able to shrink tumors by injecting THC into them. The study was conducted on lab rats with tumors. Those who were exposed to THC lived longer than those that were not. So far, it has been able to shrink tumors in the breasts, lungs, and brain.

Protects Against Flesh-Eating Bacteria. Recent studies have shown that the cannbionoids in marijuana are effective in fighting against the super-bacteria that current antibiotics cannot defend against. In effect, it can help save one's skin if it was ever to come in contact with any super-bacteria.

Can Help With Parenting. A group of women in California who call themselves "Marijuana Moms," are working to prove that smoking marijuana can make people become better parents. They claim to marijuana keeps their families together by stimulating creativity, taking your mind off stress to better focus on the kids, and to be happy, positive role models.

Can Protect Against Heart Disease. Several studies on marijuana and blood sugar levels have revealed that those who smoke marijuana are more likely to have higher levels of HDL cholesterol, which is the type of cholesterol that can protect your heart from heart disease.

Calms People With OCD. Studies on humans with OCD show that THC-based medicines can have a faster and stronger impact at slowing the symptoms of OCD faster than other types of medicine can. Studies on animals further confirmed the results.

Reduces Pain From Fibromyalgia. Fibromyalgia, a chronic pain condition that is very hard to treat, may be able to be treated with marijuana. Many patients have reported that marijuana can help relieve a handful of the painful effects at one time while prescription drugs only have a small chance a relieving pain.

Will Create Jobs. Legalized marijuana can help create more jobs in an economy that is currently lacking job options. It can open up jobs anywhere from retail positions to lab technicians. Also, it gets rid of the black market, which can bring many negative effects to a person's job search—anything from catching a felony charge to not having a built-up resume.

Can Eliminate Racism and Profiling. According to the ALCU, black people have a 3x's more chance of being arrested for marijuana than white people. This statistic infers that most police officers profile blacks based on drug use and arrest statistics. Legalized marijuana will help erase this trend of racism and profiling.

Treats Asthma. Researchers believe that the cannabinoids in marijuana can help reduce the number of coughs associated with asthma. Also, they believe that marijuana can inhibit one's airways from inflammation, which is a common symptom of asthma.

Prescription Drug Alternative. Marijuana can serve as a prescription drug alternative, which carries many benefits. Some people find it difficult to swallow pills, so being able to smoke medicine would be a good alternative. Prescription drugs also stand to have a higher abuse and accidental overdose rate, while marijuana cannot kill. It can create more jobs and people can buy it in bulk.

Combats Morning Sickness. Studies have shown that almost 100% of women who used marijuana to fight morning sickness found that it worked very well. Marijuana can also stimulate one's appetite to offset any weight loss from throwing up too much.

Hemp Oil High in Protein. Hemp oil is high in protein, making it an excellent supplement for those who need to add more protein in their diets (vegans and vegetarians) or for those who just need extra protein in their diet. It is a safe alternative to other protein supplements.

Cures Insomnia. Studies show that marijuana can cure insomnia due to the cannabinoids found in it. It can induce a deeper, longer sleep with a shorter R.E.M period and it can even improve one's breathing while sleeping. Studies show that those who used marijuana to sleep better fell asleep by one hour faster.

Can Promote Bone Growth. Recent studies show that marijuana can help prevent the onset of osteoporosis in aging adults. However, it also found that it can reduce bone growth in younger people. While the results are still inconclusive when it comes to marijuana and bone growth, the recent studies are definitely a step forward to a new breakthrough.

Treats Dermatitis. Some researchers believe that the fatty acids in hemp oil can help treat dermatitis and skin infections that cause itchy rashes although this study is still waiting on further research.

Reduces Risk of Artery Blockage. Recent studies have found that very high doses of THC can help stop your arteries from hardening. While they noted that smoking marijuana would not be enough to get the right dose of THC needed to fight artery blockage, it is possible to get enough by taking a pill-form.

Treats Psoriasis. New studies have Indicated the marijuana is effective in treating psoriasis, a skin disorder. The anti-inflammatory properties of cannabinoids are helpful in preventing flare-ups of psoriasis in some patients.

May Prevent Huntington's Disease. Early studies have Indicated that a marijuana based drug called nabilone can be beneficial in treating Huntington's Disease, a disease in which the nerve cells in the brain die. However, more research is required for conclusive results.

Can Prevent Pollen. If marijuana is grown in seedless form, it can reduce the amount of pollen in the environment. However, this can make the value of the plant go down.

Boiler Fuel. Hemp, as opposed to fossil fuels, may be used for boiler fuels. Hemp used for boiler fuel carries a value of $30 to $50 per ton. However, fuel made from hemp is a renewable resource.

Leaves Can Be Used For Mulch and Compost. The leaves of marijuana can be reused as mulch and in composts, which is giving back to the environment. Both can be used as plant fertilizers to grow more plants, therefore adding more oxygen to the planet.

Makes Granola and Birdseed. The nutrients found in hemp are often used to make birdseed and types of granola bars that are edible. Food production is a huge industry and is essential for both human and animal growth.

Makes Personal Hygiene Products. Aside from paper products, hempseed oil can also be used to create personal hygiene products, such as soaps, shampoos, bath gels, lotions, and cosmetics. Personal hygiene products that are made from hemp are more biodegradable than regular bath products and do not impact the water system as badly.

Makes Paints and Ink Products. Hemp can also be used to make paints and inks that are biodegradable, once more, better for the environment than commercial paints and inks that are manufactured. Lead and other solvents in traditional paint can damage the environment and lower air quality.

Can Be Used For Cooking Oil. Hemp oil can be used as a substitute for low-heat cooking. It gives food a nut-like taste and it serves as a substitute for olive oil when it comes to salad dressing. Hemp oil can also be used in margarine.

Makes a Great Moisturizer. Hemp oil lotions make great moisturizers because it makes your skin soft and it helps increase your blood circulation. It is perfect to use after a hot shower instead of industrial lotions.

Used in Plastics. Instead of petroleum, hemp oil can be used as the base. While petroleum can release harmful chemicals into the soil during decomposition, hemp oil has no negative impacts on the environment.

Fish Oil Substitute. Hemp oil is a great fish oil substitute because it contains similar amounts of alpha-linolenic acids, which can help fend off heart disease, depression, and arthritis.

Treats Diarrhea. The cannabinoids in marijuana positively interact with your digestive tract to help decrease pain and spasms that are related to diarrhea. Western medicine has attributed marijuana to the treatment of gastrointestinal diseases for centuries.

Lowers Crime Rate. Legal marijuana can help reduce the crime rate in areas, which lends a hand to helping public health issues in many metropolitan cities. Colorado saw a significant drop in both violent crime and property crime after the state legalized marijuana.

Treats Abdominal Pains. The cannabinoids in marijuana work positively with the digestive tract in the body to reduce inflammation, help the muscles relax, and reduce spasms that can cause ulcers, acid reflux, constipation, loss of appetite, and many other diseases and ailments that cause abdominal pains.

Eliminates Nightmares. When people enter to REM period during sleep, they are more likely to have nightmares. However, studies have shown that marijuana is able to interrupt the REM period by disturbing sleep cycles. Therefore, smoking marijuana can reduce one's likelihood of having a nightmare.

Improves Cognitive Functions. Studies show that marijuana can improve the cognitive function in middle-aged adults. Researchers interviewed participants on their drug use at age 42 and then re-interviewed them at age 50. The results showed that those who smoked marijuana showed the same or better performance on cognitive tests.

Anti-Psychotic Drug. Researchers have found that a compound in marijuana, cannabidiol, is effective at treating schizophrenia and other psychotic diseases. Studies on both humans and animals have concluded these discoveries. Cannabidiol is regarded to be just as effective as other anti-psychotic medicines.

Helps With Anger Issues. With its calming affects, marijuana can help people express their anger in a more productive and controlled manner. Marijuana also effectively treats some of the triggers of anger issues, such as sleeping problems, loss of appetite, and anxiety. Marijuana does not make people violent, rather, it helps them relax.

Treats Bipolar Disorder. Marijuana is able to treat the root causes of bipolar disorder, such as depression, suicide, and psychotic episodes. As a result, people who are diagnosed with bipolar disorder stand a better chance at controlling it.

Helps Treat Panic Attacks. Although some people believe that marijuana can cause panic attacks, it can actually help treat them. Stress, one of the main causes of panic attacks, can easily be erased with small doses of marijuana. It can help people relax and cope with big changes in their lives. It can also help offset the side effects of a panic attacks, such as vomiting.

Therapy For the Terminally Ill. Many researchers believe that marijuana use can be very therapeutic for those who are suffering from terminal illnesses. It can help prevent nausea and throwing up and it can also help them relax and live out the rest of their days painlessly.

Can Treat Anorexia. Since marijuana stimulates the human appetite, it can be used as a means to treat anorexia, a common eating disorder that affects many people each year. Mostly women suffer from anorexia but it can happen to men too. Untreated, anorexia can be fatal. If marijuana can inspire people to eat, it can ultimately save lives.

Treats Hypertension. By tackling some of the root causes, marijuana can be an effective way to treat hypertension, also known as high blood pressure. Hypertension can be caused by weight gain, stress, and tobacco use. However, marijuana does not promote any of those things. Most people who use marijuana stay away from tobacco, have a higher metabolism, and are not under as much stress.

Fights Fatigue. Marijuana can help balance the hormones in the body that can cause fatigue. It also can help induce sleep and help people sleep longer and deeper, which means they will have more energy stored up to use throughout the day.

Treats Spinal Injuries. Studies have found that the compound cannabidiol can help improve mobility in those who have spinal injuries. The compound can improve healing and can reduce the extent of the injury. Additionally, marijuana can relieve any pain that is associated with spinal injuries.

Does Not Lower IQ. In an effort to shoot down a study that suggested marijuana can lower a person's IQ, a recent study found that socioeconomic factors were to blame in IQ differences. Despite the myth that marijuana kills brain cells, it does not have any negative impact on intelligence.

No Proven Links to Mental Illness. Again, despite the myth that marijuana is dangerous and can lead to mental illnesses, studies have found that it can actually prevent mental illness, such as bipolar disorder and schizophrenia. There is no evidence that marijuana or any of the compounds found in it attribute to mental problems.

Can Be Ingested Without Smoking. Unlike many medicines, which only have one acceptable way of being taken, people have several options when it comes to using marijuana for medical purposes. It can be smoked, it can be eaten, it can be vaporized, and in some states it can be taken in pill form.

Safer Than Heroin. Marijuana is safer to use than heroin. Heroin is a depressant and can bring peoples' moods down instead of up. It is also an addicting substance and kills many people each year. The heroin black market has caused drug dealers to sell people tainted batches which are fatal right away. Heroin also causes people to lie, cheat, steal, and hurt their loved ones. Once a person is hooked on heroin, they usually have to go to a detox facility to get off of it.

Safer Than Cocaine. Cocaine can also give people a euphoric affect but it comes at a steep price. Cocaine is a stimulant that can raise a person's blood pressure and heart rate to dangerous points. It is addicting like heroin and often requires a lengthy process to get off of it.

Safer Than Alcohol. Marijuana is safer than alcohol in the sense that it is not addictive, it does not cause violence like alcohol does, and it does not cause liver damage. You will read more about how marijuana is safer than alcohol in Chapter 6.

Safer Than Designer Drugs. Marijuana is safer than designer drugs such as ecstasy or its more pure form, Molly. Drugs like these can cause peoples' bodies to overheat, dehydrate, and they can also cause significant brain damage.

Safer Than Meth. Marijuana is safer than meth in the sense that is does not cause any brain damage and it is not addictive. Meth can cause insomnia, violence, anxiety, mood swings, and confusion. Meth also increases the risk of contracting AIDS, HIV, and Hepatitis.

Chapter 4: Common Myths about Marijuana

In an attempt to keep marijuana listed as a Schedule I drug among other conspiracies, many myths and lies about marijuana have surfaced over the years. Many of these myths popped around during the 1960s and 1970s and have carried over to today. Unfortunately, this had ended in the result of having too much misinformation available about marijuana. This chapter will take a look at the 10 most common myths about marijuana, most likely the ones that you have heard from school or from your parents, and debunk each one. It is time to bring the truth about marijuana to the light!

Myth #1: Marijuana Causes Long-Term Memory Loss/Problems. While it is true that marijuana can cause short-term memory loss while it is in one's body, there is no proof that marijuana has any effect on long-term memory loss or long-term memory problems. If a person smokes marijuana, they will still remember everything they learned prior to smoking and will be able to retain information in the future. It is just difficult to remember what happens while you've got the drug in your body.

Myth #2: Science Has Proven That Marijuana is a Harmful Substance. This myth is just flat out not true. In one publication of British Medical Journal *The Lancet,* one article states, "the smoking of cannabis, even long term, is not harmful to health." Furthermore, there has been no evidence of marijuana-related deaths, no emergency room visits, and no long-term impacts.

Myth #3: Smoking Marijuana Can Cause a Decrease in Motivation. While some strains of marijuana can make you feel "lazy" or relaxed during intoxication, studies have shown that marijuana cannot cause a long-term decrease in motivation. One study tested the effects of a high-dose of marijuana on several testers over a long period of time. The results showed no reports of a decrease in motivation. Interestingly, another study also showed that people who smoke marijuana are more likely to have higher paying jobs.

Myth #4: Marijuana Use Causes Crime. Since many people are under the thoughts that marijuana use can lead to aggression, it also leads to crime. In reality, several studies have shown that marijuana users are less likely to engage in crime because it actually reduces aggression. Since many localities in which marijuana is still illegal considers possessing it a crime, many people get confused.

Myth #5: Marijuana is a Gateway Drug. Many people relive that once a person smokes marijuana, it leads them to try other, harder drugs. While studies show that hard drug users have smoked marijuana before, there are studies that compare marijuana-only users to hard drug users. That study shows that there is almost no link that connects marijuana users to hard drugs.

Myth #6: Marijuana Causes Lung Damage. Of of the most popular myths about marijuana is that it is just as harmful as tobacco use and it causes lung cancer. On the contrary, studies have shown that those who smoke marijuana verses those who smoke tobacco smoke less often, therefore limiting their exposure to smoke. Also, marijuana does not contain any harmful additives and chemicals that are put into cigarettes. Finally, researchers have found that marijuana does not have any negative effects on the lungs, such as tobacco, which can cause emphysema.

Myth #7: Marijuana is Addictive. One rumor that has floated around about marijuana is that it is highly addictive. It even ranks on the federal drug list as having a "high potential for abuse." However, studies have found that marijuana is in fact not addictive. Rather, less than 1% of the population smokes twice a day or more. While some people may find it hard to stop smoking marijuana, researchers believe that the real issue is the problem of breaking a bad habit, not an addiction.

Myth #8: Marijuana Kills Brain Cells. This myth emerged from an experiment that involved animals and marijuana. In the experiment, researchers noted structural changes that took place in the brains of the animals. Two human studies have since been looked at and has found no correlation. On the other hand, legal drugs such as alcohol can lead to damaged brain cells.

Myth #9: Marijuana is More Potent Today Than It Ever Was. Due to government studies that show differing numbers, many people believe that the potency of marijuana is higher today than it was in the 60s. This because the samples that the government used to get their statistics were stale bricks that were left in police lockers from the early '70s. The potency of most marijuana remains the same today.

Myth #10: The THC That Gets Stored in Fat Cells Can Last Up To 2 Months. While it is true that your fat cells absorb THC and marijuana can be detected in your system up to a few weeks after you smoke it, the THC remains harmless. It does not affect your brain, heart, or any other body part. However, once you come down from your high, the high is over.

Chapter 5: What Famous People Are Saying About Marijuana

Despite the fact that recreational marijuana use is still illegal in most of the United States today, many famous figures have admitted to using it and supporting it. Although some famous people, such as Justin Bieber, have recently given marijuana a bad name in the news, many famous people have given it a good name.   From former presidents to famous rappers, this chapter will take a look at what some of the most significant figures in the media are saying about marijuana.

Bill Clinton. In a 2013 interview with Fusion TV, former President of the United States Bill Clinton did not say that he ever smoked marijuana but rather said that he never denied not smoking it. Clinton has admitted to smoking marijuana during his time as a Rhodes scholar although he said that he did not inhale the smoke. He then went on to say that he never tried it after that. Clinton believes that the laws and attitudes toward marijuana use should vary from country to country, based on making the right choices. He further believes that marijuana should not be treated as a hard drug and doesn't think it will promote violence.

Snoop Dogg. Snoop Dogg, the well-know rap artist who promotes marijuana use and exposing its benefits. Snoop believes that if marijuana was legal in every state, the crime and violence rates would go down as they have in Amsterdam. Despite his multiple charges for marijuana possession, Snoop Dogg encourages marijuana use in his family. He currently smokes with his oldest son and is helping him launch his own rap career, which includes many marijuana-related songs. Snoop believes that marijuana use with his son will help keep their relationship strong and close.

Wiz Khalifa. Wiz Khalifa, another famous rap artist, is also very open about his passion for and use of marijuana. His one song, *Kush and Orange Juice* features a specific strain of marijuana and he openly admits that he "wakes and bakes." Most interestingly, he is currently producing his own brand of rolling papers and he has admitted to spending $10,000 on marijuana each month. Although he doesn't condone other people making the same marijuana-related choices as he has, he also believes that the federal legalization of marijuana could help make the world a better place.

Willie Nelson. Willie Nelson, a very well-known country singer who is currently in his 80's, has always been a big supporter of marijuana. He has recently made a reference to marijuana in the title of his latest autobiography and he has joked that it will only kill someone if a bale of it drops on it. Despite running into some trouble with the law enforcement, Nelson believes that marijuana has never taken a negative toll on his health and he has positive thoughts on its recent legalization in Washington and Colorado.

Barrack Obama. Barrack Obama, the current president of the United States, has openly admitted to experimenting with marijuana when he was younger and he has also admitted that it is not as bad as alcohol. Despite his liberal views on marijuana, he has discouraged his daughters from trying it and has said that it is a waste of time and a bad habit. Obama looks at the legalization of marijuana in Washington and Colorado in good taste and believes it should expand.

Jesse Ventura. Jesse Ventura, former governor of Minnesota, is one of the biggest advocates of legalizing marijuana state-wide. He believes it will end the war on drugs and it could save the United States $100 billion each year. Ventura believes that marijuana is the part of a culture and that addiction is a medical problem instead of a criminal problem.

Chapter 6: Death Rate Comparison—Marijuana vs. Tobacco, Alcohol, Prescription Drugs

Though there have been some crazy (and untrue) myths that people can die from smoking marijuana, marijuana has had and maintains a death rate of 0. As you know from Chapter 3, marijuana is non-addictive and it can actually benefit yourself health instead of hurting it. This chapter aims to help you forget everything bad you've heard about marijuana. The statistics even show that marijuana is safer than tobacco, alcohol, and prescription drugs, all of which are legal in all 50 states. Yet, marijuana is only legal for recreation in two states and for medical purposes in 21.

Tobacco. Tobacco, one of the main ingredients of cigarettes, causes over 443,00 deaths each year. Cigarettes are responsible for causing lung cancer, respiratory diseases, and overall damages to the lungs. Studies have found that while tobacco can decrease the speed of air that one can blow out, marijuana can actually increase it. Although studies also Indicated that heavy or long-term marijuana use could have the opposite effect, researchers noted that cigarette smokers smoke more often than marijuana smokers. It is believed that marijuana can increase the speed that one can exhale because marijuana smokers take deep inhales while smoking, which may attribute to stronger lungs.

Alcohol. According to the United States Center for Disease Control and Prevention, alcohol kills more than 37,000 people each year. Studies have named alcohol as one of the top most toxic drugs in the

United States, compared to marijuana, which is all natural and does not contain anything toxic. Alcohol increases health costs far more than marijuana does and alcohol can damage the brain. Finally, alcohol is an addictive drug. Many people all around the world suffer from the disease that is better known as alcoholism. Not only does alcohol kill people from directly drinking too much of it, but it can also cause people to fall and hit their heads, throw up and choke on their vomit, and kill themselves and others in drunk driving cases. Marijuana does not cause any of these things. Finally, while alcohol is known to cause aggression and leads to many violent crimes, marijuana causes people to relax and be peaceful.

Prescription Drugs. Prescription drugs, mostly painkillers, pose as harmful drugs despite the fact that doctors can legally prescribe them. Unfortunately, prescription drugs are addictive and although they require a prescription, doctors do not have a system to track them. Many people go "doctor-shopping" to obtain multiple prescriptions to feed their addictions. They are even available for sale on the internet, which does not require a prescription. Prescription drug overdoses account for about 45% of overdose deaths each year.

As you now know from reading chapter 3, marijuana brings more value and benefits to peoples' lives than all three of these substances combined, yet, all three of them are currently legal under federal law. While it is true that it is still illegal to possess prescription drugs for which you do not have a valid prescription, it still does not

have a significant effect on reducing prescription
drug deaths.

Conclusion: The Future of Marijuana

Although marijuana has many proven benefits on the environment, the economy, and one's health, it is still considered an illegal and dangerous drug by the federal government and by many local and state governments. However, President Barrack Obama is currently taking steps to have it removed from the Schedule I drug classification, where it is regarded as addictive and not suitable for medical use. Though many states still consider the possession of marijuana as a crime, many local governors, prosecutors, law enforcement officers, and even congressmen are gradually stepping forward in favor of legalization. In the wake of the controversy surround the legalization of marijuana, many polls and surveys have found that the majority of Americans are in favor of letting it be used for both recreational and medical purposes. Many Americans also hope that the federal government will focus more on getting treatment for current hard-drug users instead of focusing on prosecuting those who possess marijuana. Throughout the United States, many people have been banding together, holding protests, and speaking out in favor of marijuana.

At the time of this writing, the only two states to have legalized marijuana for both recreational and medical use are Washington State and Colorado. Possibly the most well-known controversy surround marijuana at this time is the ongoing argument between Colorado and New Jersey. In 2014, New Jersey Governor Chris Christie publicly slammed

Colorado's quality of life in an attempt to make his opposition to legalized marijuana known. Though New Jersey currently supports medical marijuana, the laws on recreational use and medical use for children are undeveloped. Colorado quickly came back at his quip and said that there was nothing wrong with their quality of life. The governor's delay on marijuana legislation actually caused a family to move out of New Jersey to Colorado so their sick daughter could get the medical marijuana treatment she needed. Also, although many people wrongly believe that marijuana will attribute to more violence and crime, many experts believe that it can dramatically increase the quality of life.

Right now, it looks like Washington D.C is next on the line to potentially legalize marijuana for recreational use. Rhode Island is also looking at legalization legislation along with Vermont, Oregon, New York, Nevada, Montana, Massachusetts, Maryland, Maine, Hawaii, Delaware, California, Arizona, and Alaska. Although
most of these states have legalized medical marijuana, they are looking to legalize and tax it all completely. This would prevent many people from having a ruined background and arrest record if caught with small amounts of marijuana. It would also keep the jails free and will take a burden off of the taxpayers.

Despite any governments that are still in the dust, the public is rapidly moving toward the support of marijuana, whether anybody likes it or not. Marijuana is slowly losing its place in the War on

Drugs and many states are looking at options to decriminalize marijuana at the least. Although the future of marijuana is unclear at this time, it does look like that it could have a lasting, positive impact on the world in the near future.

www.ingramcontent.com/pod-product-compliance
Lightning Source LLC
Chambersburg PA
CBHW051255170526
45165CB00004B/1725